COMPLETE 0 POINT FOOD LIST

The Complete Ingredient list Recipes and High-Point Food to Avoid

Harley W. Norman

Copyright © 2024 by Harley W. Norman

All rights reserved

No part of this publication may be reproduced, stored in a retrieval system. or transmitted. in and form or by any means, electronic, mechanical, photocopying, recording, or otherwise, without the prior written permission of the author. The information in this eBook is true and complete to the best

of our knowledge. All recommendations are made without guarantee on the part of the author or publisher. The author and publisher disclaim any liability in connection with the use of this information.

Table of Contents

Introduction 4

    Overview of the Zero Point Food Concept................................. 7

    How to Use This Guide 10

    Benefits of Incorporating Zero Point Foods into Your Diet 13

Part I: Foods to Eat 16

    Fruits 16

    Vegetables 20

    Proteins 24

    Beverages 28

Part II: Foods to Avoid 32

    High-Point Foods to Minimize 32

Common Mistakes and Misconceptions 35

    Misinterpreting Zero Point Foods as "Unlimited" 35

    Ignoring Portion Sizes 38

    Overlooking the Nutritional Quality of Foods 41

Part III: Planning and Implementing a Balanced Diet 44

Chapter 7: Creating Balanced Meals with Zero Point Foods ... 44

    Sample Meal Plans 44

    Incorporating Zero Point Foods into Your Daily Diet 47

Chapter 8: Tips for Eating Out and Social Events 50

Choosing Zero Point Foods in Restaurants 50

Managing Social Events and Gatherings 53

Conclusion 56

Introduction

In the heart of a bustling city, nestled between the aroma of freshly baked bread and the vibrant hues of the local farmers' market, Sarah found herself at a crossroads. She was a culinary enthusiast, known among her friends for her sumptuous dinners and inventive recipes. However, lately, Sarah felt that her passion for food was clashing with her journey towards a healthier lifestyle. The more she delved into diet plans and nutrition guides, the more confused and restricted she felt. That was until she discovered the "Complete 0 Point Food List" book, a discovery that would reshape her culinary world.

The book was elegantly displayed in the window of her favorite little bookstore, its cover boasting vibrant images of fruits, vegetables, and other wholesome foods. Intrigued, Sarah stepped inside, the bell above the door chiming her arrival. As she flipped through the pages, she was greeted with a beautifully organized table of contents that promised not just recipes, but a new philosophy towards eating.

The "Complete 0 Point Food List" wasn't just another diet book; it was a guide to rediscovering the joy of eating without the guilt. It introduced Sarah to an array of foods that she could enjoy without having to count calories or points. The book was meticulously structured, dividing foods into categories such as fruits, vegetables, proteins, and even beverages, all of which were considered zero-point foods. These were items she could indulge in, knowing they were nourishing her body and supporting her health goals.

What truly set the book apart, however, was its approach to the foods to avoid. Instead of listing them as forbidden, the book educated readers on making mindful choices, understanding the nutritional content of foods, and recognizing the importance of moderation. It was a holistic approach that spoke to Sarah on a personal level.

Sarah was particularly drawn to the section on planning and implementing a balanced diet. The book provided practical advice on creating balanced meals, incorporating zero-point foods into daily diets, and even tips for eating out and managing social events. It wasn't just about what foods to eat; it was about crafting a lifestyle that was sustainable, enjoyable, and liberating.

The story that unfolded in the pages of the "Complete 0 Point Food List" resonated with Sarah. It wasn't just about losing weight or following a strict diet; it was about making peace with food and embracing it as a source of energy, joy, and health. She realized that this book was more than just a purchase; it was an investment in her well-being.

As Sarah left the bookstore, book in hand, she felt a sense of excitement and anticipation. She was eager to embark on this new culinary adventure, armed with knowledge and inspiration. The "Complete 0 Point Food List" had offered her something invaluable: the freedom to enjoy food without reservation, the tools to make healthier choices, and the confidence to trust in her journey towards wellness.

For anyone standing at the crossroads of wanting to indulge in their love for food while nurturing their health, Sarah's discovery of the "Complete 0 Point Food List" serves as a testament to the possibility of finding balance. It's a story not just of a book, but of transformation, empowerment, and the joy of eating.

Overview of the Zero Point Food Concept

The zero point food concept is central to understanding how individuals can enjoy a wide range of foods without the guilt or complexity often associated with dieting and calorie counting. This innovative approach, highlighted in the "Complete 0 Point Food List," emphasizes foods that do not count towards daily point or calorie totals in specific diet plans, effectively allowing for consumption without portion size restrictions. These foods are chosen based on their nutritional profile, being high in essential nutrients while low in calories and unhealthy fats, which makes them an excellent choice for those looking to lose weight or maintain a healthy lifestyle without sacrificing the pleasure of eating.

Fruits and vegetables, with a few exceptions, generally dominate the list of zero point foods. They are rich in fiber, vitamins, and minerals, and are known for their role in promoting digestive health, reducing the risk of chronic diseases, and aiding in weight management. By making these foods zero points, the concept encourages individuals to fill their plates with nutrient-dense options, promoting satiety and reducing the likelihood of overeating high-calorie foods.

Proteins, particularly lean proteins like skinless poultry, fish, eggs, and legumes, also feature prominently on the zero point food list. These foods are crucial for building and repairing tissues, supporting immune function, and promoting a feeling of fullness. Including them as zero point foods recognizes their essential role in a balanced diet while acknowledging the importance of managing portions to support weight loss and overall health goals.

The zero point food concept also extends to some beverages, with water, black coffee, and unsweetened tea being prime examples. These drinks support hydration without adding calories, making them ideal for inclusion in a health-conscious diet. By encouraging the consumption of these beverages, the concept helps individuals avoid sugary drinks and high-calorie beverages that can hinder weight management efforts.

One of the most appealing aspects of the zero point food concept is its simplicity. It eliminates the need for meticulous tracking and measuring, making healthy eating more accessible and less daunting. This approach not only fosters a positive relationship with food but also encourages lifelong healthy eating habits by emphasizing food quality over quantity.

Moreover, the concept is designed to be flexible and adaptable, fitting into various dietary preferences and lifestyles. Whether one is a vegetarian, follows a gluten-free diet, or has other dietary restrictions, the zero point food list offers options that can be incorporated into any meal plan. This inclusivity ensures that individuals can enjoy a diverse and satisfying diet while working towards their health and wellness goals.

In essence, the zero point food concept is more than just a list of foods; it's a philosophy that champions a balanced, nutritious, and enjoyable approach to eating. By focusing on foods that can be eaten freely, it encourages individuals to make healthier choices naturally, leading to sustainable weight loss and improved health without the feeling of deprivation or restriction. The "Complete 0 Point Food List" embodies this philosophy, offering a practical guide to embracing a healthier lifestyle through mindful eating and a deep appreciation for the nutritional value of foods.

How to Use This Guide

Using the "Complete 0 Point Food List" guide is akin to embarking on a journey towards a healthier, more vibrant lifestyle without the burden of constant calorie counting or restrictive dieting. This guide is designed to empower you with the knowledge and tools necessary to make informed choices about what you eat, focusing on foods that nourish your body without adding points to your daily intake. Here's a comprehensive walkthrough on how to make the most of this guide.

First, familiarize yourself with the concept of zero-point foods. These are foods that you can eat without having to track or limit based on most diet plan guidelines. They are typically high in nutrients and low in calories, making them excellent choices for anyone looking to maintain a healthy diet. This guide categorizes these foods into fruits, vegetables, proteins, and beverages, providing you with a vast array of options to incorporate into your meals.

Next, take the time to explore the section dedicated to foods to eat. Here, you'll find an extensive list of zero-point foods, along with suggestions on how to prepare and combine them into delicious, nutritious meals. Whether you're a fan of smoothies, salads, stir-fries, or snacks, this section offers creative ideas to keep your meals exciting and satisfying.

The guide also addresses foods to avoid or consume in moderation. While the focus is on zero-point foods, understanding which foods are high in points is crucial for balancing your diet. This section educates you on identifying foods that might hinder your progress and offers tips on how to make smarter choices without feeling deprived.

One of the most valuable aspects of the guide is its practical advice on creating balanced meals. This isn't just about mixing and matching zero-point foods; it's about understanding the nutritional content of what you eat and ensuring you're getting a balanced intake of carbohydrates, proteins, fats, and fibers. The guide provides examples of balanced meals and snacks that can fit into any lifestyle, making it easier to plan your diet.

Furthermore, the guide doesn't leave you stranded when it comes to dining out or attending social events. It acknowledges the challenges of sticking to your diet in social settings and offers strategies for navigating menus, making smart food choices, and even how to indulge responsibly. This ensures that you can enjoy social gatherings without derailing your health goals.

Lastly, embrace the journey of integrating zero-point foods into your life as a long-term commitment to your health. The guide is not a quick fix but a comprehensive resource for making sustainable changes to your eating habits. It encourages you to experiment with new foods, recipes, and meal planning techniques, making the process enjoyable and fulfilling.

By following the "Complete 0 Point Food List" guide, you equip yourself with the knowledge to make healthful eating a natural part of your daily routine. It's about transforming your relationship with food, where eating becomes a source of pleasure and nourishment, paving the way for a healthier, happier you.

Benefits of Incorporating Zero Point Foods into Your Diet

Incorporating zero point foods into one's diet brings a multitude of benefits, offering a fresh perspective on healthy eating without the complexity of constant calorie counting or restrictive meal planning. These foods, typically encompassing fruits, vegetables, lean proteins, and certain beverages, are considered "free" in various diet programs because they contribute minimally to daily caloric intake while providing essential nutrients. Emphasizing these foods encourages individuals to make healthier choices, fostering a balanced approach to nutrition and weight management.

One of the primary advantages of zero point foods is their ability to promote weight loss in a sustainable manner. By filling up on foods that are low in calories yet high in volume, individuals can achieve a sense of fullness without consuming an excessive number of calories, naturally leading to a calorie deficit. This method eliminates the need for meticulous tracking, making the weight loss journey less daunting and more manageable over the long term.

Furthermore, the nutritional density of zero point foods is a key factor in their appeal. These foods are rich in vitamins, minerals, antioxidants, and fiber, which play crucial roles in maintaining overall health. For instance, the high fiber content found in many fruits and vegetables aids in digestion and can help stabilize blood sugar levels, while lean proteins are essential for muscle repair and growth. Incorporating a variety of these foods ensures a wide range of nutrients that support bodily functions, from immune defense to energy metabolism.

The psychological benefits associated with incorporating zero point foods into the diet cannot be overlooked. The flexibility offered by not having to track these foods reduces the mental burden often associated with dieting, making it easier to stick to healthy eating habits. This approach can lead to a more positive relationship with food, where choices are driven by nourishment and satisfaction rather than strict rules and restrictions. It encourages a mindset shift from eating less to eating smarter, emphasizing the quality of the food rather than just the calorie content.

Additionally, the versatility and accessibility of zero point foods make them an excellent choice for meal planning and preparation. Whether one is cooking a quick family dinner or packing a lunch for work, these foods can be easily incorporated into a variety of dishes, from salads and smoothies to stir-fries and soups. This versatility ensures that meals are not only nutritious but also diverse and flavorful, preventing dietary boredom and making it more likely for individuals to adhere to their eating plans.

Finally, zero point foods promote a more inclusive and less restrictive dietary approach, which can be particularly beneficial for social situations and dining out. Instead of navigating through a minefield of "forbidden" foods, individuals can focus on enjoying a wide array of zero point options available in most settings. This aspect fosters a sense of normalcy and ease in social interactions, eliminating the stress and isolation often felt by those following strict diets.

The inclusion of zero point foods in one's diet offers a comprehensive approach to healthy living, balancing weight management goals with nutritional needs and psychological well-being. This approach demystifies the process of eating well, making it accessible, enjoyable, and sustainable. It underscores the idea that healthy eating is not about restriction but about making informed choices that support one's health and lifestyle.

Part I: Foods to Eat

Fruits

Incorporating fruits into one's diet is a cornerstone of healthy eating, especially when adhering to a plan that includes zero point foods. Fruits, with their natural sweetness, variety of flavors, and rich nutritional profiles, are an excellent choice for anyone looking to enhance their diet without adding significant calories. The following table lists several fruits that are considered zero point foods, along with their nutritional benefits, making them an essential part of a balanced diet.

Fruit	Serving Size	Calories (Approx.)	Key Nutrients
Apple	1 medium (182g)	95	Fiber (4g), Vitamin C (14% DV), Potassium (6% DV)
Banana	1 medium (118g)	105	Vitamin B6 (20% DV), Vitamin C (17% DV), Potassium (12%

Fruit	Serving Size	Calories (Approx.)	Key Nutrients
			DV), Fiber (3g)
Berries (Strawberries, Blueberries, Raspberries)	1 cup (152g for strawberries, 148g for blueberries, 123g for raspberries)	50 (strawberries), 84 (blueberries), 64 (raspberries)	High in antioxidants, Vitamin C (149% DV for strawberries, 24% DV for blueberries, 54% DV for raspberries), Fiber (3g for strawberries, 4g for blueberries, 8g for raspberries)
Citrus (Oranges, Grapefruits)	1 medium (131g for oranges, 230g for grapefruits)	62 (oranges), 52 (grapefruits)	Vitamin C (116% DV for oranges, 64% DV for grapefruits), Fiber (3g for both)

Fruit	Serving Size	Calories (Approx.)	Key Nutrients
Kiwi	1 medium (69g)	42	Vitamin C (117% DV), Vitamin K (38% DV), Fiber (2g)
Mango	1 cup, sliced (165g)	99	Vitamin C (67% DV), Vitamin A (25% DV), Fiber (3g)
Peach	1 medium (150g)	58	Vitamin C (17% DV), Vitamin A (10% DV), Fiber (2g)
Pear	1 medium (178g)	101	Fiber (6g), Vitamin C (12% DV), Vitamin K (10% DV)
Watermelon	1 cup, diced (152g)	46	Vitamin C (21% DV), Vitamin A (18% DV), Hydration (92% water)

DV = Daily Value

These fruits are not only low in calories but are packed with vitamins, minerals, and fiber, making them an excellent addition to any meal or snack. They offer a range of health benefits, including:

- **Fiber:** Important for digestive health and helps in feeling full, which can aid in weight management.
- **Vitamins and Minerals:** Each fruit listed provides a wealth of vitamins and minerals that support overall health. For example, Vitamin C is crucial for the immune system and skin health, while potassium supports heart health.
- **Antioxidants:** Many fruits, especially berries, are rich in antioxidants, which help fight free radicals in the body, reducing inflammation and lowering the risk of chronic diseases.

Including a variety of these zero point fruits in your diet can help ensure you're getting a broad spectrum of nutrients essential for health, all while enjoying the natural sweetness and flavors that make them so appealing. Whether eaten alone as a snack, mixed into a smoothie, or used to add sweetness to dishes, these fruits are versatile and beneficial additions to any meal plan focused on health and wellness.

Vegetables

Below is a detailed table focusing on vegetables that are commonly found on the "Complete 0 Point Food List," highlighting their nutritional benefits and categorizing them based on their nutrient profile. This table serves as a guide to incorporating these zero-point vegetables into your diet effectively.

Vegetable	Type	Nutritional Information per 100g	Health Benefits
Spinach	Leafy Green	23 kcal, 2.9g protein, 3.6g fiber, high in Vitamin A & K	Supports bone health, aids in digestion, boosts immune system
Kale	Leafy Green	49 kcal, 4.3g protein, 2g fiber, high in Vitamin C & K	Promotes eye health, enhances skin and hair, aids in detoxification
Broccoli	Cruciferous	34 kcal, 2.8g protein, 2.6g fiber, rich in Vitamin C & K	Supports heart health, contributes to cancer prevention, boosts brain health

Vegetable	Type	Nutritional Information per 100g	Health Benefits
Cauliflower	Cruciferous	25 kcal, 1.9g protein, 2g fiber, contains Vitamin C & K	Aids in weight loss, reduces inflammation, supports hormonal balance
Carrots	Root	41 kcal, 0.9g protein, 2.8g fiber, high in Vitamin A & beta-carotene	Improves vision, supports skin health, aids in digestion
Bell Peppers	Nightshade	20 kcal, 0.9g protein, 1.7g fiber, very high in Vitamin C	Enhances immune function, supports healthy skin, aids in the absorption of iron
Tomatoes	Nightshade	18 kcal, 0.9g protein, 1.2g fiber, rich in Vitamin C & lycopene	Supports heart health, contributes to skin health, provides cancer-fighting antioxidants

Vegetable	Type	Nutritional Information per 100g	Health Benefits
Zucchini	Squash	17 kcal, 1.2g protein, 1g fiber, contains Vitamin A & manganese	Aids in weight loss, improves heart health, supports vision
Mushrooms	Fungi	22 kcal, 3.1g protein, 1g fiber, rich in B vitamins	Boosts immune system, supports brain health, aids in weight management
Eggplant	Nightshade	25 kcal, 1g protein, 3g fiber, contains nasunin & fiber	Promotes brain health, aids in digestion, supports heart health
Cucumbers	Gourd	15 kcal, 0.7g protein, 0.5g fiber, contains Vitamin K	Hydrates the body, supports skin health, aids in weight loss
Asparagus	Shoot	20 kcal, 2.2g protein, 2.1g fiber, high in Vitamin K & folate	Supports prenatal health, aids in weight loss, promotes digestive health

These vegetables, all considered zero points, offer a variety of essential nutrients, including vitamins, minerals, and fiber, making them invaluable for maintaining a balanced and healthy diet.

Incorporating a diverse range of these vegetables can help in achieving a variety of health benefits, from improved digestion and enhanced immune function to better heart health and weight management. The versatility of these vegetables also means they can be easily included in a wide array of dishes, ensuring a diet that is not only nutritious but also enjoyable and sustainable.

Proteins

In the context of the "Complete 0 Point Food List," focusing on proteins that are categorized as zero point can significantly enhance one's understanding of how to incorporate these essential nutrients into a diet without adding to the daily point tally.

Below is a detailed table outlining various zero point proteins, including a brief nutritional overview for each. This selection of proteins is celebrated for their minimal calorie impact and substantial contribution to daily nutritional needs, particularly in diets that prioritize health and wellness without strict calorie counting.

Protein Source	Serving Size	Calories (approx.)	Protein (g)	Fat (g)	Notable Nutrients
Chicken Breast (skinless, cooked)	3 oz	140	26	3	High in niacin, vitamin B6, phosphorus
Turkey Breast (skinless, cooked)	3 oz	125	26	1.5	Rich in selenium, vitamin B3, B6

Protein Source	Serving Size	Calories (approx.)	Protein (g)	Fat (g)	Notable Nutrients
Fish (cod, salmon, tuna, etc.)	3 oz	70-200	15-25	0.5-13	Omega-3 fatty acids, vitamin D (fatty fish)
Shrimp (cooked)	3 oz	84	20	0.3	Selenium, vitamin B12, iodine
Crab (cooked)	3 oz	84	17	1	Vitamin B12, zinc, copper, selenium
Eggs	1 large	70	6	5	Vitamin D, B6, B12, zinc
Beans (black, kidney, chickpeas)	½ cup cooked	100-120	7-8	0-0.5	Fiber, iron, folate
Lentils	½ cup cooked	115	9	0.4	Fiber, iron, folate, manganese
Peas (green)	½ cup cooked	62	4	0.2	Vitamin C, vitamin K, manganese

Key Nutritional Highlights and Benefits:

- **Lean Poultry (Chicken and Turkey Breast):** These are excellent sources of high-quality protein, which help in muscle repair and growth. The vitamins and minerals present support various bodily functions, including energy metabolism and immune system health.
- **Fish:** Offers a wide range of proteins with the added benefit of omega-3 fatty acids in fatty fish like salmon, which are crucial for heart health and cognitive function. Vitamin D in fatty fish supports bone health and immune function.
- **Shellfish (Shrimp and Crab):** Besides being lean sources of protein, shellfish are rich in minerals like selenium, which plays a key role in antioxidant defense, and vitamin B12, important for nerve function and blood formation.
- **Eggs:** Considered a complete protein as they contain all nine essential amino acids. Eggs are also a source of various vitamins and minerals, including vitamin D, which is not widely available in many foods.
- **Legumes (Beans and Lentils):** While not animal-based, these plant proteins are an essential part of a balanced diet, especially for vegetarians. They are high in fiber, which aids in digestion and provides a sense of fullness, alongside a profile rich in iron and folate.

- **Peas:** A great vegetable protein source, peas also provide a good amount of vitamins and minerals, including vitamin C, which supports the immune system, and vitamin K, which is essential for blood clotting.

This comprehensive table showcases how zero point proteins can be both versatile and nutritious, offering an array of options for those looking to maintain or improve their health through diet. Including these proteins in meals ensures that one's diet is not only balanced but also conducive to various health goals, including weight loss, muscle building, and overall well-being.

Beverages

These beverages can be consumed without impacting one's daily points allowance in certain diet plans, offering hydration and nutrition while supporting overall health goals.

This table also includes essential nutritional information for each beverage, though it's important to note that actual nutritional values can vary based on specific brands and preparation methods.

Beverage	Description	Nutritional Information per 8 oz (Approx.)
Water	The most essential zero-point beverage, vital for hydration and supporting bodily functions. Can be consumed plain, sparkling, or infused with fruits for flavor.	0 calories, 0g fat, 0g protein, 0g carbohydrates
Black Coffee	A zero-point choice when consumed without added sugar or cream. Offers a mild stimulant effect due to	2 calories, 0g fat, 0.3g protein, 0g carbohydrates, 95mg caffeine

Beverage	Description	Nutritional Information per 8 oz (Approx.)
	caffeine and contains antioxidants.	
Green Tea	A beneficial beverage rich in antioxidants, particularly catechins, which may support heart health and weight loss. Best consumed unsweetened.	2 calories, 0g fat, 0.5g protein, 0g carbohydrates, 28mg caffeine
Herbal Tea	Includes a wide variety of caffeine-free options such as peppermint, chamomile, and hibiscus, each offering unique health benefits, from digestion support to relaxation.	0 calories, 0g fat, 0g protein, 0g carbohydrates
Lemon Water	Plain water infused with lemon not only enhances flavor without adding points but also provides vitamin C and aids digestion.	6 calories, 0g fat, 0.1g protein, 2g carbohydrates

Beverage	Description	Nutritional Information per 8 oz (Approx.)
Unsweetened Iced Tea	A refreshing alternative to hot teas, can be enjoyed with a variety of tea bases like black or green, served cold without sweeteners.	2 calories, 0g fat, 0g protein, 0g carbohydrates, varies with tea base

Additional Notes:

- **Hydration:** It's important to prioritize hydration for overall health. These zero-point beverages can contribute to daily fluid intake goals.
- **Caffeine Content:** Beverages like coffee and green tea contain caffeine. While they offer metabolic benefits and alertness, it's wise to monitor caffeine intake, especially for those sensitive to its effects.
- **Nutritional Benefits:** Beyond hydration, some of these beverages offer additional health benefits. For example, green tea is known for its antioxidant properties, and lemon water can aid in digestion and provide a modest amount of vitamin C.
- **Preparation Matters:** To ensure these beverages remain at zero points, avoid adding sugar, cream, or other calorie-dense

ingredients. Opt for natural or calorie-free flavor enhancers if desired.

Remember, while these beverages are considered to have zero points, moderation is key, especially with caffeinated options. Ensuring a balanced intake of various foods and beverages is essential for maintaining a healthy and sustainable diet.

Part II: Foods to Avoid

High-Point Foods to Minimize

This guide is designed to help individuals understand why certain foods, despite being delicious, should be consumed in moderation to maintain a balanced and healthy diet.

Category	Examples	Reasons to Minimize
Processed Meats	Bacon, Sausages, Deli Meats	These foods are often high in saturated fats and sodium, which can increase the risk of heart disease and high blood pressure. Additionally, processed meats are linked to an increased risk of certain cancers. Their high point value reflects not just their caloric density but also their potential negative impact on long-term health.
High-Fat Dairy Products	Cheese, Whole Milk, Cream	High-fat dairy products are calorie-dense and high in saturated fats, contributing to increased cholesterol levels and a higher risk of cardiovascular disease. They can also contribute

Category	Examples	Reasons to Minimize
		significantly to daily caloric intake, making weight management more challenging.
Sugary Foods	Cakes, Cookies, Candy	Sugary foods are high in calories and low in nutritional value. They can lead to spikes in blood sugar levels, contributing to energy crashes, weight gain, and an increased risk of type 2 diabetes. These foods often contribute to overeating and are associated with poor diet quality.
High-Carb Foods	Bread, Pasta, Rice (Refined Varieties)	Refined carbohydrates are stripped of their fiber and nutrients during processing, leading to a faster digestion and a rapid increase in blood sugar levels. This can result in hunger cues shortly after consumption, potentially leading to overeating. Additionally, high intake of refined carbs is linked to increased risk of obesity and metabolic syndrome.

This table highlights the importance of moderating the consumption of high-point foods in a diet that prioritizes zero point foods. By understanding the reasons behind minimizing these foods, individuals can make informed decisions that align with their health and wellness goals, without feeling deprived or restricted. The focus should always be on a balanced diet that incorporates a variety of nutrients to support overall health.

Common Mistakes and Misconceptions

Misinterpreting Zero Point Foods as "Unlimited"

Misinterpreting zero point foods as "unlimited" is a common pitfall that can derail individuals from their health and wellness goals. While zero point foods are an integral component of a balanced diet, promoting the consumption of fruits, vegetables, lean proteins, and certain beverages without the need to track each item's point value, it's crucial to approach these foods with mindfulness. The designation of zero points is meant to encourage healthier eating choices, not to imply that these foods can be eaten in boundless quantities without any repercussions.

Firstly, even though zero point foods are typically lower in calories and high in nutrients, consuming them in excessive amounts can still lead to caloric surplus. For instance, fruits, while packed with vitamins, minerals, and fiber, also contain natural sugars. Overconsumption can contribute to a higher caloric intake than anticipated, potentially slowing down weight loss progress or leading to weight gain. Similarly, lean proteins are essential for muscle repair and growth, but they are not calorie-free. Large portions can significantly increase daily caloric intake.

Moreover, the concept of unlimited zero point foods can overshadow the importance of variety and balance in a diet. Relying too heavily on these foods might lead to nutritional imbalances or deficiencies in the long run. For example, neglecting whole grains, nuts, and seeds because they have point values might deprive the body of essential fatty acids, antioxidants, and other nutrients vital for overall health.

Another aspect to consider is the psychological impact of viewing zero point foods as unlimited. This perception might foster an unhealthy relationship with food, where the focus shifts from eating for nourishment and enjoyment to eating because "it's free." It can disrupt cues of hunger and satiety, leading individuals to eat more out of perceived permission rather than actual need, which is counterproductive to developing mindful eating practices.

Additionally, the misinterpretation of zero point foods as unlimited could lead to missed opportunities for learning about portion sizes and the nutritional content of foods. Understanding how to gauge portions and the impact of various food choices on health and well-being is crucial for maintaining a balanced diet and achieving long-term health goals.

In essence, while zero point foods play a pivotal role in facilitating healthier eating habits without meticulous tracking, it's essential to consume these foods mindfully. Recognizing that they are part of a comprehensive dietary approach—one that emphasizes variety, balance, and moderation—is key to navigating the journey toward health and wellness successfully. Embracing zero point foods as a means to enrich the diet rather than viewing them as free-for-all can pave the way for sustainable eating habits and a healthier relationship with food.

Ignoring Portion Sizes

Ignoring portion sizes is one of the most common pitfalls individuals encounter when incorporating zero point foods into their diet. The allure of these foods is evident; they are nutritious, can be consumed without tracking every bite, and are deemed "free" in the context of certain diet plans. However, this freedom can sometimes lead to the misconception that these foods can be eaten in unlimited quantities without any consequences. While zero point foods are indeed healthier choices, understanding and respecting portion sizes is crucial for a balanced diet and successful weight management.

One of the key reasons portion control is essential, even with zero point foods, is that calories still count. For instance, while fruits and vegetables are packed with vitamins, minerals, and fiber, they also contain calories. Consuming large amounts of these foods without mindfulness can lead to a caloric surplus, which may hinder weight loss efforts or even lead to weight gain. This is particularly true for starchy vegetables and certain fruits with higher sugar content.

Moreover, disregarding portion sizes can also distort one's understanding of hunger and satiety cues. Eating large quantities of food in one sitting, even if they are zero point foods, can lead to overeating habits. It's important to listen to one's body and eat until satisfied, not stuffed. This practice encourages a healthier relationship with food, where eating decisions are based on physical hunger rather than the perceived freedom to eat without limits.

In addition, ignoring portion sizes of zero point foods can overshadow the importance of dietary variety. A well-rounded diet includes a balance of macronutrients - proteins, fats, and carbohydrates - and micronutrients from a wide range of food sources. Focusing too much on consuming large amounts of zero point foods might limit the intake of other essential nutrients found in foods with points or calories, potentially leading to nutritional imbalances or deficiencies.

For those following a diet that features zero point foods, it's advisable to enjoy these foods in reasonable portions. This approach supports a sustainable eating pattern that can be maintained long-term, beyond any structured diet plan. It also helps in cultivating mindfulness about eating habits, encouraging individuals to make intentional choices about what and how much to eat.

While zero point foods are a valuable component of a healthy diet, it's important to remain mindful of portion sizes. Respecting portion sizes ensures that the diet remains balanced, supports weight management goals, and promotes a healthy relationship with food. Remember, the goal is to nourish the body, satisfy hunger, and enjoy the wide range of flavors and textures that these foods offer, all while maintaining a sense of dietary freedom and flexibility.

Overlooking the Nutritional Quality of Foods

Overlooking the nutritional quality of foods is a significant oversight that can occur when individuals rely heavily on the zero point food list as part of their diet strategy. While these foods are an excellent choice due to their low calorie count and ability to be consumed in relatively unrestricted quantities, focusing solely on zero point foods without considering their overall nutritional value can lead to an imbalanced diet.

Zero point foods are typically selected because they are lower in calories and higher in nutritional density, which encourages their consumption. However, not all zero point foods are created equal in terms of what they offer nutritionally. For example, while fresh fruits and vegetables are packed with vitamins, minerals, and fiber, they may not provide sufficient protein or healthy fats, which are crucial for overall health. This can lead individuals to inadvertently neglect important food groups or nutrients that are essential for maintaining energy levels, muscle function, and overall bodily functions.

Another aspect of this issue is that it can lead to a skewed perception of what is healthy. Just because a food is labeled as zero points does not necessarily mean it should be the main focus of one's diet. This misconception might cause people to consume large amounts of certain foods, like fruits, while avoiding higher-point foods that contain healthy fats and proteins, such as avocados and nuts. These foods play a critical role in a well-rounded diet by providing essential fatty acids, sustained energy, and satiety, which can aid in weight management and overall health.

Moreover, the focus on zero point foods alone might result in missing out on other nutritious foods that, although they carry points or calories, have health benefits that zero point foods do not provide. For instance, whole grains and legumes are not typically zero point foods, but they offer dietary fiber, protein, and a range of micronutrients that are vital for digestive health and maintaining stable blood sugar levels.

This oversight can also lead to an excessive intake of certain types of zero point foods, such as those high in natural sugars or certain types of vegetables that, when consumed in vast amounts, might contribute to digestive issues or an excessive intake of certain nutrients. Balance and moderation are key, even when foods are considered zero points.

It is essential for individuals to remember that a healthy diet is a balanced one that includes a variety of foods from all food groups. Incorporating zero point foods should be seen as a way to enhance dietary options without restrictions, but not at the expense of nutritional completeness. Understanding the full nutritional content of foods, including those with points, helps in making informed decisions that support a healthy lifestyle.

The best approach is to use the zero point food list as a flexible guide rather than a strict rulebook, combining these foods with nutrient-dense foods that have points to ensure a balanced intake of carbohydrates, proteins, fats, and other essential nutrients. This strategy ensures that the diet remains varied and nutritionally adequate, promoting long-term health and wellness.

Part III: Planning and Implementing a Balanced Diet

Chapter 7: Creating Balanced Meals with Zero Point Foods

Sample Meal Plans

Crafting meal plans that integrate zero point foods effectively ensures a diet rich in nutrients while also supporting weight management and overall health. By focusing on a variety of fruits, vegetables, lean proteins, and whole grains, individuals can enjoy satisfying, balanced meals. Below are sample meal plans that highlight how to incorporate these foods into daily eating patterns, emphasizing the importance of balance and variety.

For breakfast, a vibrant start to the day could include a bowl of mixed berries (strawberries, blueberries, raspberries) topped with a dollop of non-fat Greek yogurt and a sprinkle of cinnamon. This meal combines the natural sweetness and antioxidants of berries with the protein-rich yogurt, providing energy without added sugars or fats. For those who prefer a savory start, scrambled egg whites with spinach, tomatoes, and mushrooms offer a filling, protein-packed option rich in vitamins and minerals.

Lunch could be a colorful salad composed of leafy greens like arugula and spinach, topped with slices of grilled chicken breast, a variety of vegetables such as bell peppers, cucumbers, and carrots, and a dressing made from lemon juice and herbs. This meal is low in calories but high in fiber and protein, ensuring satiety until the next meal. Alternatively, a vegetable soup with lentils provides a comforting, nutrient-dense option, combining the hydrating properties of soup with the fiber and protein of lentils.

Dinner might feature baked salmon seasoned with herbs and lemon, served alongside steamed broccoli and cauliflower, and a quinoa salad with diced cucumbers, tomatoes, and a splash of vinegar for dressing. This meal is balanced with lean protein, complex carbohydrates, and a variety of vegetables, supporting muscle repair and providing essential nutrients. For a plant-based option, a stir-fry with tofu, a medley of vegetables (such as zucchini, bell peppers, and snap peas), and a side of brown rice can offer a satisfying and nutritious end to the day.

Snacks throughout the day can include whole fruits like apples or pears, carrot and celery sticks with hummus, or a small handful of mixed berries. These options are not only low in calories but also provide a good mix of fiber, vitamins, and minerals, making them perfect for staving off hunger between meals.

Beverages throughout the day should focus on hydration without added calories. Water, herbal teas, and black coffee are excellent choices. Infusing water with slices of lemon, cucumber, or berries can add a refreshing twist for those seeking variety.

Incorporating zero point foods into meal planning doesn't mean restricting flavor or variety. Instead, it encourages a creative approach to eating that focuses on nutrient density, balance, and the pleasure of enjoying whole, unprocessed foods. These sample meal plans are designed to inspire, demonstrating that a diet centered around zero point foods can be both delicious and nourishing.

Incorporating Zero Point Foods into Your Daily Diet

Incorporating zero point foods into daily meals is a strategy that can transform one's approach to healthy eating, making it more flexible and enjoyable while still aligning with nutritional goals. These foods, which typically include fruits, vegetables, lean proteins, and some beverages, offer a way to add volume, fiber, and essential nutrients to meals without adding significant calories. This approach encourages a focus on whole, nutrient-dense foods, facilitating weight management and overall health without the need for strict calorie counting.

A balanced meal that includes zero point foods can provide a satisfying mix of protein, carbohydrates, and fats, along with vitamins and minerals, to support bodily functions and sustain energy levels throughout the day. For breakfast, one might start with a base of zero point foods such as eggs and mixed berries, adding a whole grain slice of toast and avocado for healthy fats and additional fiber. This combination ensures a hearty, balanced start to the day, incorporating proteins, healthy fats, and carbohydrates.

Lunch and dinner can follow a similar pattern, where half the plate is filled with zero point vegetables, a quarter with lean protein such as chicken breast, fish, or beans, and the remaining quarter with whole grains or starchy vegetables that may carry points but are essential for a balanced diet. For instance, a lunch plate could feature a large salad with various vegetables, grilled chicken, and a side of quinoa or a whole grain roll. This not only adheres to the principle of incorporating zero point foods but also ensures a well-rounded intake of macronutrients.

Snacks are another opportunity to include zero point foods in the diet. Instead of reaching for processed snacks, one can opt for fruits, vegetables with hummus, or a small portion of nuts for those on programs where certain nuts are considered zero points. These choices keep hunger at bay with nutrient-rich options, preventing overeating at mealtimes.

Incorporating zero point foods into meals also encourages culinary creativity. Exploring different herbs and spices can add variety and flavor without the need for calorie-dense sauces or dressings. For example, roasting vegetables with garlic and rosemary, or seasoning fish with lemon and dill, can make zero point foods the highlight of any meal.

It's important to remember that while zero point foods can and should form the foundation of a healthy diet, they work best in conjunction with a variety of other foods. Including whole grains, healthy fats, and even occasional treats ensures a diet that is both nutritionally complete and sustainable long-term. This approach allows for flexibility and personalization, making it easier to stick to healthy eating habits without feeling restricted.

Lastly, hydration plays a critical role in a balanced diet, and incorporating zero point beverages like water, herbal teas, and black coffee helps to maintain hydration levels without adding calories. These beverages can also contribute to the feeling of fullness and overall well-being.

Incorporating zero point foods into daily meals is a practical and enjoyable way to create balanced, nutrient-dense meals that support health and wellness goals. This approach not only aids in weight management but also enhances the overall quality of the diet, making healthy eating a sustainable and pleasurable part of everyday life.

Chapter 8: Tips for Eating Out and Social Events

Choosing Zero Point Foods in Restaurants

Eating out and attending social events can often feel like navigating a minefield for those trying to maintain a healthy diet, especially when following a plan that includes zero point foods. The temptation of rich, indulgent dishes can be overwhelming, but with a strategy focused on zero point foods, dining out can remain an enjoyable and guilt-free experience. Here are some tips for making healthier choices that align with the zero point food philosophy when eating away from home.

Start with a plan. Before heading to a restaurant or event, review the menu online or consider the type of food that will be available. Identify dishes that are likely to include zero point foods such as fruits, vegetables, lean proteins, and whole grains. This pre-planning can help you make informed decisions and avoid feeling overwhelmed by the menu choices.

Look for grilled, baked, or steamed options. These cooking methods are less likely to add unnecessary calories from oils or butter that are often used in frying or sautéing. Dishes that highlight these cooking techniques are more likely to be centered around zero point foods, such as grilled chicken or fish, steamed vegetables, and baked potatoes (with the skin, for the added fiber).

Ask for modifications. Don't hesitate to request changes to your meal that align it more closely with your dietary goals. This could mean asking for dressings or sauces on the side, substituting a high-point side dish with a salad or steamed vegetables, or requesting that your meal be prepared with less oil or butter. Most restaurants are accommodating to such requests, and these small changes can make a big difference in aligning your meal with zero point food choices.

Focus on salads and broth-based soups. These dishes can be great ways to incorporate zero point foods into your meal, especially if they are loaded with vegetables and lean proteins. However, be mindful of additions like croutons, cheese, and creamy dressings or soups, which can quickly elevate the point value of these seemingly healthy options. Opting for vinaigrette dressings on the side or clear soups can help keep your meal within the zero point range.

Incorporate fruits and vegetables whenever possible. Whether it's choosing a side of fruit instead of fries, adding extra vegetables to your pizza, or opting for a vegetable-based dish, increasing the proportion of fruits and vegetables in your meal can help you fill up on zero point foods. This not only enhances the nutritional value of your meal but also aligns with the principle of eating more foods that are nutrient-dense and lower in calories.

Share or skip high-point items. If you're tempted by a dish that doesn't align with zero point foods, consider sharing it with someone else at your table. This allows you to enjoy a taste without overindulging. Alternatively, if there's a high-point appetizer or dessert that's particularly tempting, consider skipping it altogether and focusing on the healthier options you've selected.

Stay hydrated. Drinking water throughout your meal can help you stay hydrated and feel more satisfied. Sometimes thirst is mistaken for hunger, leading to unnecessary eating. Keeping a glass of water handy and sipping on it throughout your meal can prevent this confusion and support your decision to focus on zero point foods.

By incorporating these strategies, dining out and attending social events can remain enjoyable experiences that don't derail your health goals. Choosing zero point foods in these settings encourages a flexible, balanced approach to eating that supports wellness without sacrificing social interactions or the pleasure of eating out.

Managing Social Events and Gatherings

Managing social events and gatherings while adhering to a diet that incorporates zero point foods requires planning and strategies that can help individuals enjoy themselves without compromising their nutritional goals. Social settings often present a range of tempting foods that may not align with the zero point food list, making it a challenge to stick to a healthy eating plan. However, with thoughtful preparation and mindful choices, it is entirely possible to navigate these events while maintaining a balanced diet.

One effective strategy is to eat a small, nutritious meal or snack before attending any social event. Choosing foods from the zero point list, such as fruits, vegetables, or lean proteins, can help curb hunger and reduce the temptation to overindulge in high-calorie or high-point foods that are commonly served at parties. This preemptive approach allows individuals to feel satisfied, not starved, which leads to better decision-making at the buffet table.

When at the event, it's helpful to survey all the food options before starting to fill a plate. Identify which dishes are likely made from zero point foods and prioritize these. For example, salad greens, fresh fruits, and grilled vegetables typically fit within this category. By filling up on these healthier options first, there's less room on the plate and in the stomach for higher-point items, effectively controlling overall intake.

Another tip is to bring a zero point dish to share. This ensures that there will be at least one item that aligns with one's dietary goals, and it also introduces others to the concept of delicious, healthful eating without points. Dishes like a vibrant vegetable platter with a zero point dip, a fresh fruit salad, or a lean protein like shrimp cocktail are usually well-received and complement any spread.

When it comes to beverages, it's best to stick with zero point options like water, herbal teas, or black coffee. Alcoholic and sugary drinks can add a significant number of points and calories. If choosing to indulge, opt for a glass of wine or a light beer, and limit consumption to help maintain dietary goals. Staying hydrated with water throughout the event can also help manage hunger and maintain clear decision-making.

Engaging in conversations away from the food tables is another helpful tactic. By focusing on social interactions rather than the food available, one can reduce mindless eating. Enjoying the company of others can be just as fulfilling as enjoying the meal and helps emphasize that the event is about socializing, not just eating.

Lastly, it's important to be flexible and kind to oneself. If deviations from the diet plan occur, it should not be seen as a failure. Social events are a time to celebrate, and occasional indulgences are part of a balanced life. The key is to enjoy these moments mindfully and then return to regular healthy eating habits without guilt.

By applying these strategies, managing social events and gatherings while following a diet plan that includes zero point foods can be both enjoyable and successful. These tips help maintain focus on health goals without sacrificing social engagement, making it possible to navigate any social setting with confidence.

Conclusion

The journey through understanding and integrating the Complete 0 Point Food List into daily life is an empowering approach to healthy eating that emphasizes freedom, flexibility, and the enjoyment of food. This method allows individuals to focus on consuming foods that nourish without the burden of meticulous calorie counting, offering a refreshing perspective on diet and wellness that supports long-term health benefits.

Key to this approach is the notion that eating well doesn't have to be restrictive or overwhelming. By prioritizing zero point foods, which include a wide array of fruits, vegetables, lean proteins, and selected beverages, one can enjoy satisfying, nutritious meals that support weight management and overall health. These foods, rich in essential nutrients, help form the foundation of a balanced diet, promoting improved digestion, enhanced immune function, and increased energy levels.

Moreover, understanding the importance of moderation even within the zero point food categories ensures that the diet remains balanced and sustainable. Learning to listen to the body's cues for hunger and fullness, and respecting portion sizes, plays a crucial role in maintaining a healthy relationship with food. This awareness prevents the common pitfalls of overeating and nutritional deficiencies, fostering a holistic view of health that transcends simple dietary changes.

Additionally, the ability to navigate social events and dining out without deviating from health goals shows the practicality and adaptability of incorporating zero point foods into any lifestyle. It encourages social interactions and personal enjoyment without the guilt typically associated with dieting, demonstrating that a balanced approach to eating can coexist with a vibrant social life.

Incorporating zero point foods into one's diet is not just about making healthier food choices; it's about making a commitment to a healthier life. It's about recognizing that each meal is an opportunity to positively impact one's health and well-being. The Complete 0 Point Food List is more than just a guide—it's a tool that empowers individuals to take control of their eating habits, enjoy their food, and embrace a lifestyle that values nutrition and health without compromising flavor or satisfaction.

Ultimately, the journey with the Complete 0 Point Food List is ongoing and evolving. It requires persistence, consistency, and a willingness to adapt to personal needs and circumstances. It's a testament to the fact that a healthy diet can be as rich and fulfilling as it is nourishing and beneficial. This approach not only supports physical health but also enhances the quality of life, proving that what we eat profoundly impacts our overall well-being. Embracing this comprehensive and thoughtful way of eating ensures that each choice at the dining table is a step towards a healthier, happier future.

Made in the USA
Coppell, TX
06 July 2024